The big secret about stress is that what appears to be causing stress—the *stressor*—is seldom what causes damage. It is how you *respond* to what is happening that does that. Make stress work *for* you rather than against you—change your response to stress—and you can turn negative into positive. This has been demonstrated again and again in objective quantitative research. The implications of these findings are simple: if you can meet stress as a challenge and if you can also eliminate as many unnecessary stressors as possible from your life, you can not only make a positive experience of stress but also protect the long-term health of your body and have a lot of fun in the process.

By Leslie Kenton
Published by Ivy Books:

BEAT STRESS
BOOST ENERGY
GET FIT
LOOK GREAT
LOSE FAT
SLEEP DEEP

BEAT STRESS

Leslie Kenton

Ivy Books
Published by Ballantine Books
Copyright © 1996 by Leslie Kenton

http://www.randomhouse.com

Library of Congress Catalog Card Number: 96-94972

ISBN 0-8041-1719-5

Manufactured in the United States of America

First Canadian Edition: June 1997

10 9 8 7 6 5 4 3 2 1

Contents

Author's Note

The material in this book is intended for information purposes only. None of the suggestions or information is meant to be prescriptive. Any attempt to treat a medical condition should always come under the directions of a competent physician. Readers should always consult with a health care professional before starting a new diet or exercise program. Neither the publisher nor I can accept responsibility for injuries or illness arising out of a failure by a reader to take medical advice. I am only a reporter. I also have a profound interest in helping myself and others maximize our potential for positive health.

BEAT
STRESS

Introduction

We worry about stress, speculate about stress, and wish it would go away. Seldom do we stop to ask what it is. Little wonder. For stress is a complicated thing even to define. The word *stress* comes from the language of engineering, meaning "any force that causes an object to change." In engineering the specific change caused by stress is known as strain, and there are four possible kinds—torsion, tensile, compression, and shearing. In human terms the strain is your body's response to physical, chemical, emotional, or spiritual forces, asking in some way that you adapt to them. The idea that stress is all bad is patent nonsense. Stress can be the spice of life, the exhilaration of challenge and excitement, the high of living with heavy demands on you. And, like the tempering process involved in the production of a piece of good steel, once you make a friend of stress, forces that once seemed to be working against you become positive energies that define you, strengthen you, and help you express your own brand of creativity and joy.

For the big secret about stress is that what appears to be causing stress—the *stressor*—is seldom what causes damage. It is how you *respond* to what is happening that does that. Make stress work *for* you rather than against you—change your response to stress—and you can turn negative into positive. This has been demonstrated again and again in objective quantitative research. The implications of these findings are simple: if you can meet stress as a challenge and if you can also eliminate as many unnecessary stressors as possible from your life, you can not only make a positive experience of stress but also protect the long-term health of your body and have a lot of fun in the process.

Stress and relaxation are like two sides of a coin. Learn to move easily from one to another and you will begin to experience your life as a satisfying and enriching challenge like the ebb and flow of the tides. Then you will never again have to worry about getting stuck in a high-stress condition that saps your vitality, distorts your perceptions, and can even lead to premature aging and chronic illness.

The secret of getting the right balance between stress and relaxation is threefold.

- First, take a look at the kind of stress that is part of your life, eliminate unnecessary stressors, and discover new ways of working with the others.

- Second, learn one or more techniques for conscious relaxation and practice them until they become second nature.

- Finally, explore ways of expanding your mind, honoring your individuality, and creating an environment that supports both.

Not only will this help your body stay in balance and increase your level of overall vitality, but it can also bring you a sense of control over your life that is hard to come by any other way.

CHAPTER 1

Get the Balance Right

Fight or Flight

Human beings are natural seekers of challenge. In primitive times the challenge was one of survival, and this gave a certain rhythm to the working of the body. When in danger from some external cause—say, a wild animal—the body reacted instantaneously, providing the energy resources to fight or flee. The physiological changes brought about in the body by stressors are described as the *fight or flight mechanism*. Adrenal secretions flash into the blood. The pulse races, blood pressure increases, and breathing speeds up. Within seconds the body's full energy potential is realized, so one can deal effectively with the threat—either by fighting

and destroying it or by running away to safety.
Both actions use up all the chemical by-products
of the stress reaction—the sugar, the adrenaline, and the increased muscle strength that
accompanies them. When the danger passes,
the body relaxes. The production of adrenaline
slows to a trickle, and heart rate and breathing
decrease. The body returns to its vegetative
rhythm, restoring normality to physiological
processes and bringing a sense of mental and
physical well-being.

Our bodies still react to danger in the same
way, but now our sense of danger comes from
different threats—the pressure of deadlines at
work, the fear that someone is trying to take
your job from you, or worry about losing the
person you love most if you do what *you* really
want to do. All these and many others cause
someone to move into the danger rhythm state
without suffering physical or mental damage.
The trouble is that modern life, with its noise,
quick pace, social pressures, environmental
poisons, and orientation to sedentary mental
work, presents many of us with almost constant
threat situations. This is particularly true in
the business world where some people, instead
of moving rhythmically out of the danger state
into the vegetative one, remain for long periods (in some cases every waking hour) in the
danger state with all the internal physical con-

ditions that accompany it. Sooner or later, unless they move out of the threatening situation, the predator who at one time preyed on the wild beast will begin to prey internally on them.

Getting the Balance Right

The automatic, or involuntary, functions of your body are governed by the autonomic nervous system. It looks after the changes in the rate at which your heart beats. It regulates your blood pressure by altering the size of veins and arteries. It stimulates the flow of digestive juices and brings on muscular contractions in the digestive system to deal with the foods you take in. It makes you sweat when you are hot and is responsible for the physical changes in your body that come with sexual arousal. This autonomic system has two opposing branches: the *sympathetic* and the *parasympathetic*.

The sympathetic branch is concerned with expansiveness and energy expenditure—particularly the energy involved with stress and meeting challenges. The other branch of the autonomic nervous system—the parasympathetic—is concerned with *rest* and regeneration rather than action. The workings of the parasympathetic branch are more or less in opposition to those of the sympathetic branch. The parasympathetic branch slows your heartbeat, reduces the flow of air to your lungs, stimulates the digestive system, and helps relax your muscles.

When you are in a state of stress, the sympathetic nervous system has precedence over the parasympathetic. When you are relaxed, the parasympathetic branch is dominant. A good balance between the two is the key to stress-wise living as well as a door to enormous energy and continuing health. Unfortunately, few of us get it right by accident; we have to learn.

Instead, there is the dynamic person who is ever seeking greater challenges and heights of personal achievement and who seems to have endless energy—until he discovers a few years on that he is suffering from high blood pressure and is told either to ease up or to go into long-term drug therapy for hypertension. At the other extreme is the gentle, quiet, sensitive person who luxuriates in physical comforts, dreams beautiful dreams, and impresses everyone with his serenity but who never seems able to put any of his ideas into effective action. The first person is what is known as a *sympathetic-dominated* person. The second is called *para-sympathetic-dominated*. To make the most of your potential in the world and still remain well enough and receptive enough to enjoy the fruits of your labors, you want to be neither—or both.

Making Stress Work for You

Begin by taking a look at how you may be putting yourself under *unnecessary* stress. Try to identify unnecessary stressors in your life. By eliminating as many as you can you free a lot of energy for more positive use and for meeting important challenges. For instance, physical inactivity is a stressor—it decreases your body's ability to function at optimum levels, it encourages the storage of wastes in the muscles and skin, and makes you chronically fatigued. So instead of indulging in it, start some kind of exercise program—swimming or running or dancing—and follow it regularly three or more times a week. Many people who take up regular exercise report that they experience conceptual shifts so that things that appeared stressful before no longer bother them.

Like cigarettes and drugs, various foods and drinks can be heavy stressors, too. They offer nothing in the way of positive health and vitality but are a constant drain on the adaptive energy in your body. It is well established that caffeine, alcohol, tobacco, sugar, and excess fat are stressors. Not only are they substances your body doesn't need, but they also actively work against the body's normal, healthy functioning.

Many emotional stressors can also be discarded. Take a look at what continues to trigger the stress response in your life and ask yourself whether you really want to meet this challenge—for instance a relationship that doesn't work or a job you hate—or whether it is something that prevents you from turning a lot of your creative energies to more constructive use. Some stressors provide challenges from which one can grow. Others are simply habitual. They lead nowhere and bring little in terms of increasing awareness or ability to make better use of life.

You might want to start a journal in which you record observations and feelings about your own life. Take a look at the work you do and ask yourself if you find it really satisfying. Are the financial responsibilities you have taken on really necessary? Can you reduce them in any way? You might just try having the courage to drop some of them and accept the changes this will bring about.

Each of us needs not only to face up to the demands of stress but also to take responsibility for removing it wherever it is no longer useful and relevant to us. Are you one of those miracle-working superhumans who work from nine to five—or six or seven—and then come home to look after home and family and relatives and friends? Do you do the shopping, errands, and feeding of partner or children and still expect yourself to emerge from it at the end of the day a scintillating wit? This is what I call playing the superhuman role—a role that is commonplace among creative and ambitious people. It is a dangerous game to play.

Push yourself to your limits and you could produce physical symptoms such as headaches; colds and flu; back, neck, or shoulder ache; chronic fatigue; and PMT, or emotional troubles ranging from feelings of inadequacy to depression, irritability, and dependence on alcohol or drugs. You could also find you were not doing the best at your job or for the people closest to you either, even though you may actually have been sacrificing your own needs to theirs. Many an intimate relationship has failed as a result of the superhuman syndrome. Don't let it happen to you.

Write It Out

At this point I suggest you make a list of everything you think of as a stressor in your life—work, relationships, financial commitments, family—anything that causes you to feel stressed. Now make yourself a chart and write each of these stressors in the left-hand column. Think carefully about each one and decide whether it is possible to drop that stressor altogether, to change it in some way, or to embrace it—to turn it from a negative object of fear into a challenge. For instance, if you have too many financial commitments, can any of them be eliminated? If you have cable or satellite television, could you do without it? What would the consequence be? Perhaps you would find you suddenly have much more time for yourself—to read more, visit friends, spend time relaxing. If your work is a stressor, is there anything you can do to change it, or better still, can you embrace it as a challenge? If you are eating too much fat, sugar, and white flour, decide to make an effort to alter your diet.

In the meantime take a look at these general guidelines and see if you can apply any of them.

- **Stop doing everything yourself.**
  Start delegating both at work and at home and, whenever you can, get someone else to do what needs to be done.

- **Reach for the top but never struggle in vain.**
  Take a close look at your values. What really matters to you? You can't have everything. Make choices. Otherwise you could end up a workhorse who's ultimately not very good at anything.

- **Don't say yes to everything.**
  When something is asked of you, give yourself

time to consider the request before you immediately agree. Is it something you can handle with relative ease? What are you going to have to lay aside to do it? What is it going to cost you in terms of time?

- **Forget the hero image.**

  You are only human. And you'd be surprised how much pleasure it can bring to other people when they feel they can do something for you for a change. Express your needs and many of them are likely to be satisfied. Lock them away behind the perfectly together superhuman image you project and you go it alone.

- **Guard your time jealously.**

  Limit the time you spend on inessential things such as seeing people you don't really care about seeing just because you feel it is expected of you. Cut back on the chores you feel you have to do. Do you really have to? Could somebody else do them for you? Or could they remain undone for the sake of your peace of mind?

- **Sort your priorities.**

  Take a look at what is absolutely essential to your life and what is marginal. If you can, write these things down on a piece of paper, then make sure the time and effort you spend on each thing is in line with these priorities. Take an active role in deciding how you will spend your time and live your life. Don't just let it happen.

- **Create a routine.**
  From day to day you need to make sure you
  have time to relax and take care of yourself and
  time to spend with the people you love. Recre-
  ation and having fun are as important as hard
  work, responsibility, and success. Make sure
  you get the balance right.

CHAPTER 2

Eat Well

One of the things that most subjects your body to negative stress is eating the wrong kinds of food. This has to be the most common stressor in almost everyone's lives and the one we can most easily do something about. The shelves of supermarkets and the tables in restaurants are full of tasty and seductive dishes that do little to strengthen your body's ability to handle stress positively. Most of these foods are made from refined flour and contain additives and preservatives. The typical packaged, ready-in-a-minute meal is high in hidden fats, food additives, and sugars. They all put your body under stress.

Fat Chance for Freedom

Eating more fats than your body needs or eating the wrong kind of fats causes stress damage. Too much fat prevents your body from making efficient use of carbohydrates and can encourage the development of diabetes. Excess fat raises fat, cholesterol, and uric acid levels in your blood, all of which can contribute to the development of gout, arthritis, and arteriosclerosis. A high-fat diet plays an important part in premature aging and degenerative illnesses as well.

There are two kinds of fats, both of which you need to watch carefully if you want to be stress-wise: saturated and unsaturated. Saturated fats in milk products and meat are pretty useless except as a way of laying down more fat on your belly and hips. Eat a lot of saturated fats and you undermine health and leanness. The rest— unsaturated fats—are found in processed oils or in margarines and convenience foods. Most have been chemically altered so your body cannot use the essential fatty acids they once contained, leading to fatty-acid deficiencies. Such deficiencies have now become widespread in the West despite our taking in almost half of the calories we eat in the form of fats.

You do not *need* to spread your bread with butter or pour lots of oil on your salads. A diet made up of at least 75 percent vegetables, beans and legumes, fruits, and unrefined grains plus a few fresh seeds or nuts is the basis of stress-wise nutrition. Eaten with a little lean meat or fish if you like but without added oil, cheese, or butter, it will give you all the fat you need to stay healthy—a mere 15 to 20 percent of your daily calories. More than this subjects your body to unnecessary stress. Yet the average Westerner gets an amazing 45 percent of his calories from fats—far too much for long-term health.

Don't Sugar Your Blood

Sugar also comes under the stress-wise ax. By now it is common knowledge that the consumption of refined sugar has been linked with the development of degenerative illnesses. Sugar, the end of a complex refining process that takes away every vitamin, mineral, and trace of natural fiber from the beets or cane from which it is made, is a food virtually empty of nutritional benefit—except for calories. Eating sugar tends to raise your blood-sugar level and puts stress on your pancreas, challenging it to maintain normal blood-sugar levels. Sugar can also contribute to the development of arteriosclerosis. Yet most of us eat about two pounds a week of the stuff. In fact, about 20 to 25 percent of our daily calories in the West come from it. Unless sugar is eaten naturally—that is, the way you find it in a piece of fresh fruit—it is very hard on your body. It can make you tired, depressed, and emotionally unstable due to the insulin resistance the raised blood-sugar level triggers in your body. It also leads to deficiencies in the B-complex vitamins and to an imbalance in important trace minerals.

Refined carbohydrates, such as white flour, white rice, and products made from them, are not much better. They don't put your body under stress as much as sugar and excess fats do, but they have been stripped of natural fiber, which is important for detoxifying your body and protecting you from weight gain and the development of degenerative disease.

Junk the Coffee

One of the best things you can give up to improve your ability to handle stress is coffee. Just a few cups a day can both undermine your well-being and encourage you to age long before your time. Coffee contains caffeine and caffeine is a drug. One of the xanthine group of chemicals, it stimulates the central nervous system, pancreas, and heart as well as the cerebral cortex—which is why, when you drink it, you feel temporarily more alert. Some studies show, however, that while coffee drinking makes you think you are being more efficient, in reality it may impede your mental performance. Every time you drink a cup of coffee you are getting between 90 and 120 mg of caffeine. A cup of ordinary tea yields 40 to 100 mg, cocoa or cola drinks 20 to 50 mg. If you drink two to eight cups of coffee a day, you are getting a dose of the drug that any pharmacologist would reckon considerable.

Recent studies have also linked habitual coffee drinking to many stress disorders and certain mental illnesses—from quite simple depression and anxiety to overt psychosis. Also interesting is the effect on the body when you stop drinking coffee. For coffee, if you are a steady "user," is addictive. Its removal can cause powerful withdrawal symptoms. These usually appear as nausea or a headache that lasts from a few hours to several days, depending on the seriousness of the addiction and how finely tuned your system is. But the withdrawal symptoms are short-lived and worth going through to be rid of caffeine once and for all.

Go Light on Protein

The idea that you need to eat meat to stay healthy is also untrue. Studies show that a mixed diet of roots, grains, vegetables, and fruits is a much better source of high-quality protein than are the traditional meat, fish, and dairy products, which are high in fat and too concentrated in protein. Eat meat, fish, and game by all means if you want but in small quantities (100 grams, or 3 to 4 ounces a day) instead of as the main food in a meal. Or eat them only occasionally. Try to make sure it is *really* lean meat, too, such as venison, for instance, or wild boar. And remember that the vegetables you eat contain a good quantity of protein, as do beans and legumes. Eat them together with grains for high-grade protection. A bowl of bean chili eaten with a piece of corn-bread will give you the full complement of all the essential amino acids without the excess fat. You need not eat flesh foods at all if you prefer.

Until recently our need for protein has been grossly exaggerated. Most of us in the West get far more than we need. Your body needs the constituents of protein—amino acids—to build muscle, make new hormones, and carry out its metabolic processes, such as growth and the repair and maintenance of body tissue. But too much protein leaches precious minerals and trace elements, such as zinc, calcium, magnesium, iron, and chromium, from bones and tissues. These minerals are not only essential to your health, including the maintenance of firm skin and shining hair, but also to your emotional well-being.

Carbs Are King

Another common assumption that stress-wise eating challenges is the idea that you must not eat too many carbohydrates because "starches are not really good for you." Carbohydrates are the best thing you can eat for physical and emotional balance, provided, of course, they are complex carbohydrates—unrefined grains, beans and legumes, and vegetables and fruits eaten in as natural a state as possible. Starches such as brown rice or whole wheat, which have not been milled to death and deprived of most of their natural vitamins, minerals, and fiber, when taken together with fresh vegetables provide a steady stream of energy.

Clean Up

The first step to using food as a means of enhancing your body's ability to handle stress is to detoxify your body. When you eliminate foreign substances from your blood, organs, glands, and tissues—the prime purpose behind a detox—you begin to feel balanced and clearheaded. The look of your skin improves, your energy levels are increased, and your body starts to return to a healthy homeostasis.

Every minute 300 million cells in your body wear out and need to be replaced. A spring-clean diet—even for a few days—is a great beginning. The second step to being stress-wise with food is equally important. To maintain the new feeling of well-being after your body has been internally cleansed, you might want to exchange some of your careless eating habits for new ones that provide your system with everything it needs for strength and balance, as well as very little of what it *doesn't* need. Experience this for yourself by carrying out a three-day detox to spring clean your body and balance any excess acidity from high stress by alkalinizing your system. Then you can begin stress-wise eating as the basis of a whole new lifestyle.

Go Raw

The basis of the best cleanup diet is fresh raw food, because a diet of mostly raw fruits and vegetables can spring clean the body from the inside out. It helps dissolve and eliminate toxic materials and stored wastes that have formed in various parts of the body, clear out the digestive system, restore a good acid/alkaline balance to the cells, and generally stimulate the proper functions of organs and tissues. It puts you through a kind of transformation that leaves you sparkling with vitality and feeling centered, rested, and able to tackle high-energy demands with ease. Physicians and biochemists have found that raw-food diets have curative properties that no one has yet fully explained. A Swedish scientist has discovered that health-giving substances occur in raw foods that he believes may even be capable of enhancing the genes passed on from parents to children. The notion that a diet of raw food can significantly improve your health and enhance your body's ability to deal with stress is not a new one: Ancient physicians used raw-food diets for healing.

You can use such a cleanup diet in another way, too: Every few months you can always go back to it for a few days to revitalize yourself whenever you feel you need it, perhaps at the changing of the seasons—particularly at the end of winter and at the beginning of autumn.

The Spring Clean Diet

Breakfast

Bircher muesli (pages 27–28)
or
Yogurt energy blend (page 28) plus a piece or
   two of fresh fruit or a glass of fresh fruit
   juice, if desired

Mid–morning

A glass of green drink (see the section on green
   foods on pages 32-33) made with fresh vegetable juice, fruit juice, or spring water

Lunch

Appetizer—choose from a slice of melon, avocado vinaigrette, or a bowl of clear consommé
Large salad of raw vegetables
A baked potato with low-fat cottage cheese, or a
   small bowl of brown rice, or 1–2 slices of
   whole-grain bread or toast
A piece of fresh fruit

Lunch is designed in such a way that you can
eat your spring-clean meal at a restaurant as
easily as at home. Here are some suggestions
for a packed lunch.

A large salad (undressed) in a Tupperware container

Salad dressing taken separately (if you pre-dress your salad it will go soggy)

A hard-boiled egg or some nut/seed mix

A slice or two of whole-grain crispbread

A piece of fresh fruit

Mid–afternoon

A glass of green drink made with fresh vegetable juice, fruit juice, or spring water

Dinner

Bircher muesli

A slice of toasted whole-grain bread with a little honey or sugarless fruit jam

Drinks

On a high-raw-food diet you may not be thirsty because the foods themselves have not been dehydrated by cooking and are therefore rich in organic fluids. Don't drink water with your meals but drink six to eight big glasses a day between meals. The spring-clean diet eliminates coffee, tea, soft drinks, and alcohol. Drink fresh vegetable and fruit juices, spring water (carbonated or plain), vegetable broth, and herb teas instead. The trick to making good cups of herb tea is first to find several herbs or herb combinations that you enjoy and then add one or several of the following:

A squeeze of lemon juice or a slice of lemon.

A teaspoon or so of lightly scented clear honey such as acacia or clover.

A drop of skim milk (especially nice with spicy teas).

A dash of cinnamon.

Try making a strong pot of your favorite tea and adding a sliced peach to it. Sweeten with honey, then chill for a couple of hours and drink iced in tall glasses.

HERB TEAS	
Peppermint	For settling an upset stomach
Lemon verbena or lemon grass	Good tonics
Chamomile	Calms the nerves
Goldenrod (*Solidago*)	A diuretic for those who retain water
Lime blossom or passionflower	Good for relaxation
Comfrey	Cleanses the body of toxins

Recipes

Nut/seed mix

Chop equal quantities of three or more kinds of the following nuts and seeds (choose from hazelnuts, almonds, Brazil nuts, walnuts, sunflower seeds, pumpkin seeds, and sesame seeds) in a coffee grinder, blender, or food processor. Keep the mixture in the fridge and use it for muesli or sprinkle it over salads.

Bircher muesli

- 1 apple
  squeeze of orange or lemon juice
- 2 heaped tablespoons oat flakes and 1 tablespoon raisins, soaked in $1/2$ cup of water for a couple of hours (best done overnight)
- 2 heaped tablespoons plain natural yogurt
- 1 tablespoon nut/seed mix
- 1–2 teaspoons molasses or honey to sweeten, if desired

Grate the apple and sprinkle with orange or lemon juice to prevent it from oxidizing. Stir in the soaked oat flakes and raisins. Top with yogurt and sprinkle with the nut/seed mix. Dribble a little honey over the top and serve.

You can create wonderful variations on the

muesli theme so that it never becomes boring by replacing the apple with another fruit such as a pear, banana, pineapple, berries, or mango or by mixing two or more fruits together. You can even make it with dried fruit that has been soaked overnight in water to plump it up.

Yogurt energy blend

Soak a handful of dried fruit in a bowl with enough water to cover overnight. Select unsulfured sun-dried fruits such as prunes, sultanas, raisins, peaches, pears, apricots, and dates. Blend the fruit with a cupful of plain yogurt and a dash of real vanilla essence in a blender and serve in a tall glass. Or, if you don't have time to soak the dried fruit, blend a banana with the yogurt instead and add a little honey and a pinch of nutmeg or cinnamon.

Salads

A salad is nothing less than a symphony of color and flavor that makes a meal in itself. Add together combinations of vegetables (leaf lettuce, chicory, watercress, white and red cabbage, carrots, radishes, fennel, mushrooms, red and green peppers, romaine lettuce, endive, scallions, cucumber, celery, Jerusalem artichokes, tomatoes, avocados, kohlrabi, etc.), sprinkle with seeds, nuts, chopped egg, or a little grated cheese, and toss with a delicious dressing. It can be the beginning of a whole new way of eating. Here are a couple of suggestions to get you started.

Apple slaw

1 cup white cabbage, finely chopped
1 apple, diced
1 carrot, diced
1–2 sticks celery, diced
    a few raisins and a few pecans or walnuts

Combine all the ingredients and dress with an egg mayonnaise to which has been added a teaspoon of whole-grain French mustard and a little water to thin.

Country salad

1 cup leaf lettuce, shredded
½ red pepper
1 little red cabbage, shredded
1 or 2 tomatoes, diced
    a few mushrooms, diced
2 scallions, chopped

Combine the ingredients in a bowl and dress with a French dressing with plenty of basil and a little garlic.

Special spinach salad

  a handful of spinach leaves (de-stalked), finely shredded
  a few radishes
1 avocado, diced
2 tomatoes, chopped
1 small beet, grated (optional)
1 hard-boiled egg, finely chopped

Toss all the ingredients together and dress with a tangy dressing. Try adding a teaspoon of curry powder to your ordinary French dressing and blending it with a fresh tomato.

The Stress–Wise Diet

Having completed your detox you may well find that the appeal of sugar, junk foods, tea, and coffee has waned. Now is the time to learn to get into the habit of eating wisely to handle stress. A stress-wise diet is quite naturally low in calories. Thanks to its low fat content it allows you to eat as much as you like without gaining weight. Unlike sugar, refined cereals, and breads, the unrefined grains, fruits, and vegetables are slowly digested and assimilated. They provide your body with continuous energy throughout the day, eliminating blood-sugar problems and helping you avoid fatigue.

The stress-wise approach to nutrition may at first seem a very different way of eating from what you are used to—eliminating the sweets, white flour, and large quantities of meat and gravy. But it is fairly simple to learn to cook foods without lots of fats as well as eliminating sugary foods and refined flour. And if you make the changes slowly week by week you will soon get used to beans, legumes, and grains. Whether you embrace the whole antistress way of eating or simply adjust your usual way of eating to bring it more in line with the stress-wise dietetic principles, within only a few weeks you will discover that you are on to something good. Try it and see.

Vegetable Vitality

What's so special about vegetables? Plenty. They have powerful health-enhancing properties, which is why diets high in fresh vegetables are recommended as protection against degenerative diseases such as cancer, arthritis, and arteriosclerosis. Important, too, is making sure that a good proportion of your vegetables is eaten raw. Fresh vegetables are also a rich source of natural fiber, vitamins, and minerals.

Treasures from the Sea

Seaweeds can be helpful in enhancing your body's ability to handle stress. All seaweeds— from kelp and dulse to the Japanese nori and kombu—are rich in the minerals that your body's metabolic processes require to function properly. Since convenience foods are greatly depleted in minerals and trace elements, the use of plants from the sea becomes more and more important.

Green Glorious Green

When you hear the word *green*, you naturally conjure up images of Friends of the Earth and rain forests. Sizzling with power, green can also help clean up your body and protect it in the future from the damage caused by a high-energy lifestyle. Many of the raw green foods— spirulina, chlorella, green barley, and alfalfa, for instance—are wonderful detoxifiers. They, too, help cleanse the body at a deep level and eliminate toxic wastes such as heavy metals. Green foods are rich in minerals to help rebalance the body's metabolic processes—impaired as a result of our factory-farmed, processed foods that deplete the minerals and micronutrients on which our metabolic machinery depends.

Freshwater algae such as spirulina and chlorella as well as freeze-dried young green plants such as alfalfa, wheat grass, and barley are all carefully prepared to preserve the living properties of raw foods. The Japanese call them "wonder foods" for they are packed with minerals, amino acids (which your system fairly soaks up the moment you swallow them), and—most important of all—enzymes, the very stuff of life itself. Scientists once believed that all enzymes were destroyed in the stomach when you ate raw foods. Now we know that this is not so—instead, many are taken through into the system to set your skin's and body's energetic molecules in motion, helping to create clearer, fresher skin, more vitality, and heightened resistance to stress. For while the physical by-product of stress tends to be acid, green foods alkalinize your system. This restores balance and creates a feeling of being centered and calm during highly demanding times.

For some people, they take a bit of getting used to. In time you may come to like them so much that you don't even bother to mix these green powders with fruit or vegetable juice but drink them stirred into spring water.

Stress–Wise Eating	Stress–Foolish Foods
Fresh vegetables and fruits	Refined sugar and flour and products made from them
Fresh vegetable juices	Highly processed foods and ready-made meals
Natural unsweetened low-fat yogurt—especially goat's milk yogurt	Preservatives, additives, artificial flavoring, coloring, stabilizers, emulsifiers, etc.
Fermented foods—natural sauerkraut (for instance)	Alcohol, coffee
Whole-grain breads, pasta, and cereals	Excess fat, excess protein
Beans and lentils	Most ready-made packaged cereals
Green foods such as spirulina, chlorella, green barley, alfalfa, and seaweeds	Fruit sodas, colas, diet sodas and drinks

Stress–Wise Eating

A typical day on the stress-wise diet:

On rising

A cup of hot water to which the juice of half a
lemon has been added to help alkalinize your
system and promote good elimination

Breakfast

An orange or half a grapefruit. A bowl of homemade low-fat yogurt
or
A bowl of oatmeal made from steel-cut whole
oats, with sliced banana and cinnamon on
top, and skim milk
or
Bircher muesli made with low-fat yogurt
Herb tea (or coffee substitute)

Mid–morning, if desired

Green drink
or
A piece of raw fruit
or
Some sticks of raw vegetables such as carrots or
celery

or

A slice of whole-grain bread on its own or spread
    with nonfat cottage cheese and sprinkled with
    red pepper

Lunch

A bowl of homemade vegetable or lentil soup,
    made without fat
A large salad made from raw vegetables such as
    lettuce, chicory, watercress, green and red
    peppers, celery, cauliflower, peas, sprouted
    seeds or grains, with a non-oil salad dressing,
    such as a yogurt dressing, or sprinkled with
    lemon juice

Mid-afternoon, if desired

Same as mid-morning

Dinner

A 112 g or 4 oz piece of chicken roasted without
    the skin (the skin contains lots of fat)
or
A 112 g or 4 oz piece of poached fish served
    without sauce but with a wedge of lemon
As many steamed vegetables without butter or
    sauce as you like, such as spinach, broccoli,
    cauliflower, Brussels sprouts, carrots

A bowl of steamed brown rice

A green salad with 1 tablespoon olive oil and lemon dressing (or try low-fat yogurt and crushed fresh herbs)

A whole-grain roll or two without butter

A glass of wine, if desired

Fresh fruit

CHAPTER 3

Chill Out

We live in a world of constant activity. It is a world of striving and goals, of planning and remembering—a world of never-ending sensory stimulation, ideas, and discoveries. Yet amid all this activity somewhere inside you is a center of stillness—a wordless, formless space—the home of your self or your soul. There seeds of creativity are sown that later become your ideas and your accomplishments. There in the silence and the darkness you can begin to listen to your own inner voice. You can come to know the difference between what you really want, feel, and think, and what has been programmed into you by habits, false notions, and other people's values. Locating this center within yourself, recognizing its value, and living your life more and more from it makes you a stress-hardy person. It is also an essential part of staying well. The key that opens this particular door for most of us is *relaxation*.

Passive Awareness

By relaxation, I don't mean sleeping, or flopping down on a bed when you feel you can't go on, or losing yourself in a mindless state in front of the television—although sleep is certainly essential and the other two states have things to recommend them, too. I mean something far more: learning to move at will into a state of deep stillness in which your usual concerns, your habitual thoughts, and the never-ending activity of your daily life are replaced by alert—yet totally passive—awareness. Dipping into such a state even for a few minutes allows many of the physiological changes normally experienced during sleep to take place while your body and mind are revitalized. But it is different from sleep, for while your body is passive, your mind is highly alert.

Most of us have a fear of letting go, thinking that if we give up control of things we won't be able to think clearly and independently or work well, or that someone is likely to put something over on us. In fact, just the opposite is true.

When you are able to enter a state of deep relaxation at will, this frees you from patterns of living and thinking to which you tend to be a slave—although usually an unconscious one. It enables you to think more clearly and simply and to act more directly when action is called for. The freedom that comes with this holds within it the magic for transforming negative stressors into exhilarating challenges.

Relax

Relaxation is also the most important key to mitigating the damaging effects of long-term stress. By now this has been well established scientifically. Many studies have been made of people who have been taught a relaxation technique and then were monitored as to the psychological and physiological changes that take place after fifteen or twenty minutes of practicing it. These studies show that relaxation techniques bring the parasympathetic branch of the autonomic nervous system into play, calming you, reducing oxygen consumption, lowering blood lactates (high lactate levels are associated with anxiety, arousal, and hypertension), slowing your heartbeat significantly, and changing brainwave patterns. They have also shown that repeated practice can lead to improved memory, increased perceptual ability, and a subjective feeling in participants that their work and their lives are more creative and more rewarding than they were before.

Herbert Benson, M.D., a Harvard professor and expert in behavioral medicine, did the first studies into the effects of Transcendental Meditation many years ago. He has since continued to investigate this state of psychophysical relaxation and has shown that each of us has what he calls the "relaxation response"—a natural ability to experience the relaxed state with all its benefits. All we need to tap into it is a method to turn it on. The possibilities are many. They include meditation, yoga, breathing exercises, zazen, silent repetition of a word, and autogenic training to steady aerobic exercise and biofeedback. Some will work better for you or be more enjoyable than others. It is worthwhile to try a few different techniques until you discover which ones you prefer.

Discipline for Freedom

We live in an age when discipline is often looked down upon as something that interferes with spontaneity and freedom—something old-fashioned and stifling to life. We tend to rebel against it. But the kind of discipline needed for daily practice of meditation or deep relaxation tends—far from stifling one's ability to be involved in the spontaneous business of life—actually to free it. This is something you will have to find out for yourself. At first it may take a little effort to get up fifteen or twenty minutes earlier each morning to practice a technique and to take fifteen minutes out of your busy afternoon or early evening to practice again, but you will find it is well worth it. The most common excuse is that you don't have time. The reality of the situation is that practicing twice a day for fifteen to twenty minutes will *give* you time, not take it from you, for you will find that you do everything with greater efficiency and enjoyment, and that far less of your energy is wasted on fruitless activity. Studies show that every minute you spend in a deeply relaxed state yields a fourfold return in the energy you have in your outer life.

Benson's Relaxation Response Technique

Herbert Benson, who wrote *The Relaxation Response* and *Maximum Mind*, discovered that measurable physical benefits accrue from practicing any form of meditation that depends on the silent repetition of a mantra—a word-sound. This can be done by repeating any word over and over while the eyes are closed and the body is in a quiet state.

Meditation using a mantra has a long tradition. Some mantras are said to be sacred words that have particular sound vibrations that transmit particular powers. Each tradition has its own mantras, such as *Guru Om, Om mani padme hum, La ilaha illa 'lla*, or, in the Catholic religion, *Hail Mary, full of grace, the Lord is with thee*. Whether their magic aspects are true or not, the technique works beautifully to replace the habitual chatter that runs through one's mind, the worries about things past and things yet to come.

Benson suggests you find a word that is pleasing to you. It could be anything, say, *flower*, *peace*, or *love*. He likes the word *one* as it is simple and has the connotation of unity about it. Here's how.

- Find a quiet place where you won't be disturbed for fifteen to twenty minutes and a comfortable chair that supports your back.

- Sit down and close your eyes. Give yourself a moment to settle in and you are ready to begin.

- Simply sit there, feet on the floor and eyes closed, quietly repeating your word over and over to yourself: "one . . . one . . . one . . ."

- Whenever your mind wanders or you are disturbed by a sound or thought, simply turn your mind gently back to repeating the word again.

- That is all there is to it. After 15 to 20 minutes, stop repeating the mantra and get ready to open your eyes.

- Open your eyes, stretch, and go about your everyday activities. This is a particularly useful technique once you have practiced it a few times because you can do it in so many different places, such as in a waiting room or on a commuter train or bus.

Yoga

The meaning of the word *yoga* is "union," or in modern terms, "integration." Practicing yoga regularly can bring a sense of calmness, poise, and detachment that eliminates the negative effects of stress and clears away tensions that stifle the full expression of your individuality—intellectually, emotionally, physically, and spiritually. Yoga works, through the body, to restore balance by removing energy blocks and chronic tensions.

Here is a series of simple postures that anyone can do at home even without previous experience of yoga. They will give you a feel for what yoga is all about and help you decide whether it is something that will be useful to you. In the process they can also help you sleep better, deal better with stress, and improve your overall physical condition. They are safe for anyone who is in reasonably good condition and not suffering from a slipped disk, but if you have any doubts, consult your doctor first. The secret of success is perseverance. Repeating them day after day is what brings the real rewards.

Asanas

Everyone has two kinds of energy, male and female. Male energy is like the sun—invigorating, stimulating, creative, and powerful. The male postures in yoga call forth this dynamic energy and release it.

Female energy is recuperative, calming, nurturing, and gentle. The female postures are restoring to body, mind, and spirit. Yoga attempts to release male and female energies and ultimately to fuse them in union—to integrate the person.

The first four postures are male. They are done standing and they revitalize you. The last four are female and calming. In order to achieve the best balance and effect, it is best to do them in the order given.

Do each posture slowly and deliberately, taking note of how your body feels with every movement. Never hold a position if you feel real strain, but do expect to feel some initial discomfort as your body stretches and loosens. The discomfort will pass.

Revitalizing stretcher

Stand with your hands at your sides, palms open, feet together so you are well balanced. As you inhale slowly, raise your arms above your head until your palms come together. Exhale, keeping the arm position, and rise up on your toes. Now inhale again; be aware of the stretch in your spine. Hold your breath for a few seconds. Now exhale slowly, bringing your arms down to the starting position and coming down from your toes. Repeat this three times. This exercise is particularly good to do when you get up, since it stimulates the whole system and gets you ready for the day.

Shakedown

Standing with your feet a comfortable distance apart, start the exercise by shaking your hands loosely from the wrists as vigorously as you can, then work up the arms and shoulders, shaking them too until you are shaking your whole body vigorously. Then lift up one leg at a time and shake it, too. The idea is to shake throughout the whole musculature of the body and get rid of all excess tension. The whole process should take about twenty seconds. This exercise is fun to do and its invigorating effect lasts a long time afterward.

Thigh stretcher

Standing with your hands on your hips, your heels together and toes apart in a V shape, inhale slowly, at the same time rising up on your toes. Exhale slowly, coming all the way down to a squatting position and keeping your back straight. Inhale and come up very slowly, pushing down on the balls of your feet. (It helps to keep your eyes fixed on something steady to balance.) With feet flat on the floor, exhale again, resting in the standing position. Repeat three times. This exercise tones the thigh muscles and the ankles, as well as improving your poise and balance.

Windmill

Stand with your feet about three feet apart, arms hanging loosely at your sides. Inhale, raising your arms to clasp your hands above your head. Exhale, bringing arms down, with hands still clasped, in a circle to one side and then right down toward the floor. Go around three times in each direction, inhaling on the upward swing, exhaling as you come down. Feel the twist in your torso at the side each time you start another circle as you exercise muscles not normally used. Finish by bending forward from the waist and letting the arms and torso hang loose, imagining that all the tension in your body is draining to the floor. This exercise loosens your spine and trims your midriff.

Knee touches

Lying on your back, inhale, bringing one knee up to your chest. Exhale and bring your forehead up to meet your knee. Return to the starting position without inhaling again until you raise the other knee to repeat the movement. Repeat the exercise until you have exercised each knee three times. This exercise is particularly good if you suffer from digestive problems.

Double contractions

Do the preceding exercise with the same breathing pattern as before, but pulling up both knees at once and lifting your head to meet them with

your forehead. Finish by rocking back and forth
on your back like a rocking chair. Go through
the routine six times. This loosens up the spine
and the muscles deep in the back as a preparation for more advanced postures.

Tummy twists

Lying flat on your back on the floor with your
arms spread wide to each side from the
shoulder, inhale, bringing knees up, feet flat on
the floor. Keeping knees together, exhale, twist-
ing to the right and lowering knees to the floor,
keeping shoulders flat and head straight. Hold
for ten seconds, breathing normally through
the nose. Then inhale, bringing knees back up
again slowly, and exhale, this time lowering
them to the left. Do the exercise twice, alter-
nating from side to side. This posture stretches
and brings back blood to the intestines, improves lumbar back conditions, and promotes a
strong spine, as well as tightening stomach
muscles and stretching the sides of your body
down to the hips.

The corpse

Lying on your back with your arms at the sides
of your body, palms facing upward, let your feet
fall open and your body go completely limp.

Close your eyes. Take four deep breaths through your nose, saying to yourself, "As I breathe in I take in healing energy, and as I breathe out I breathe out all the tension and all the anxiety and all the pain and negativity from my body." Now gently direct your thoughts to your feet and be aware of them. Tell them to relax and free them of all their tension. Move up slowly and gently, directing your ankles to relax, then your legs, your thighs, your hips. Let them sink heavily into the floor. Then concentrate on your spine, letting each vertebra go one after another, then the neck, head, face, eyes, and on through the shoulders, arms, hands, across the abdomen, and chest. Become aware of the feeling of complete overall relaxation and stay in this state for thirty seconds to one minute (longer if you can). This posture is an excellent way to begin and to end a session of yoga.

Autogenics

A thorough, comprehensive, and highly successful technique for relaxation and de-stressing at the very deepest levels, autogenic training was developed in the early 1930s by the German psychiatrist Johannes H. Schultz. It consists of a series of simple mental exercises designed to turn off the "fight or flight" mechanism in the body and turn on the restorative rhythm associated with profound psychophysical relaxation and in doing so, layer by layer, to gently and gradually clear away stress that you have been carrying around for many years. It is a method that when practiced daily brings results that can be comparable to those achieved by serious Eastern meditators, yet it is particularly appealing to the Western mind. For unlike many forms of meditation and yoga, autogenics has no cultural, religious, or cosmological overtones and requires no special clothing or unusual postures or practices.

Freedom to be

Schultz was a student of the clinically oriented neuropathologist Oskar Vogt, who at the turn of the century at the Berlin Neurological Institute was deeply involved in research on sleep and hypnosis. Vogt remarked that some of his patients who had been subjected to conventional forms of hypnosis soon developed the ability to put themselves in and out of a hypnotic state—or rather autohypnotic, since it was self-induced. He noticed that these patients experienced remarkable relief from tension and fatigue and also tended to lose whatever psychosomatic disorders they had been suffering from. Schultz drew on Vogt's observations and went on to design techniques allowing individuals to induce this deep mental and psychological relaxation at will.

Schultz noticed that people entering the auto-hypnotic state experience two specific physical phenomena: The first was a sensation of heaviness in their limbs and torso, and the second a feeling of diffuse warmth throughout the body. The warmth is the result of vasodilation in the peripheral arteries, and the sensation of heaviness is caused by deep relaxation in the body's muscles. Schultz figured that if he taught people to suggest to themselves these things were happening to their bodies, he could rapidly and simply introduce them to the state of what he called *passive concentration* that characterizes the autohypnotic state and that exercises great positive influence over the autonomic nervous system to restore imbalances from prolonged stress.

Heaviness and warmth

To help his patients induce the autogenic state, Schultz worked first with the sensations of heaviness and warmth. He then added suggestions about regularity of heartbeat and gentle quiet breathing—two more natural physiological characteristics of relaxation—and went on to the sensation of abdominal warmth and coolness in the forehead. These six physiologically oriented directions—heaviness and warmth in the legs and arms, regulation of the heartbeat and breathing, abdominal warmth and cooling of the forehead—became the core of autogenic training and are known as the Autogenic Standard Exercises. A person learning autogenic training goes through each of the six steps, one by one: "My arms and legs are heavy and warm, my heartbeat is calm and regular, etc.," each time he practices. Because of the body's and mind's ability with repetition to slip more and more rapidly into the deeply relaxed yet highly aware autogenic state, the formula becomes increasingly shortened until, after a few weeks or months of practicing, a state of profound psychophysical relaxation can be induced at will. And once the exercises have been mastered they can be practiced anywhere—even sitting on a bus.

Be here now

There are two important aspects to making autogenic training work for you. The first is that when doing autogenic training you accept that certain things for the moment cannot be changed. You simply let them be for the time being—right now. For it is only through acceptance that we open the gateways to change. The second important thing about autogenic training is self-discipline. You need to make time to do the exercises each day and to establish a routine—especially for the first four weeks, during which the exercises need to be done three times a day. It takes about five or ten minutes at a time to run through autogenic training while you are learning it.

The basic exercises are simple. Taking up one of three optional postures—sitting slumped rather like a rag doll on a stool, lounging in an easy chair, or lying on your back with your arms at your side—make sure you are reasonably protected from noise and disturbances and that your clothes are loose and comfortable. Generally speaking it is easiest to learn lying flat on a floor or on a very firm bed. Then, once you have got the exercise under your belt, you can do it sitting up or even very discreetly on a bus on the way to work. If you like you can record the autogenic exercise on tape and play it to yourself in the beginning, although I generally find it better to learn it very simply from the words below. Here's how.

Lie down on your back in bed or on the floor and make yourself comfortable. Close your eyes gently. Take a deep slow breath and pause for a moment. Now exhale fully and completely. Allow yourself to breathe slowly and naturally. Feel your body sinking back into the mattress or floor. Then repeat the following phrases to yourself slowly and allow yourself to feel the heaviness and warmth as you do.

The first phrase is: "My left arm is heavy ... my left arm is heavy ... my left arm is heavy ... my right arm is heavy ... my right arm is heavy ... my right arm is heavy ..." Allow yourself to let go of any tension in your arms as you say to yourself: "My left arm is heavy ... my left arm is heavy ... my left arm is heavy ..." repeating each suggestion three times. Continue to breathe slowly and naturally, remembering to exhale fully. Say to yourself: "Both arms are heavy ... both arms are heavy ... both arms are heavy." Let go of any tension in your arms.

Then say: "Both legs are heavy ... both legs are heavy ... both legs are heavy ..." As you continue to breathe slowly and naturally, say to yourself: "Arms and legs heavy ... arms and legs heavy ... arms and legs heavy ... arms and legs warm ... arms and legs warm ... arms and legs warm ..." Feel the warmth flow through to your arms and legs as you say to yourself: "Arms and legs warm ... arms and legs warm ... arms and legs warm ..."

Continue to breathe slowly and freely while you repeat silently to yourself: "My breathing calm and easy . . . my breathing calm and easy . . . my breathing calm and easy . . . my heartbeat calm and easy . . . my heartbeat calm and easy . . . my heartbeat calm and easy . . ." Feel your strong, regular heartbeat as you say these words to yourself.

Continue to breathe easily and say to yourself: "My solar plexus is warm . . . my solar plexus is warm . . . my solar plexus is warm . . ." Feel the muscles in your face relax as you say to yourself: "My forehead is cool and clear . . . my forehead is cool and clear . . . my forehead is cool and clear . . ." Enjoy the feeling of softness and calm throughout your body and say to yourself: "I am at peace . . . I am at peace . . . I am at peace . . ."

When you have finished the exercise you are ready for the return that will bring you back to normal everyday consciousness. Quickly clench both fists, take a deep breath in, flex both arms up in a stretch, then breathe out slowly and completely, returning your arms with un-clenched fists to your sides. Open your eyes. Lie for a moment with your eyes open and just allow yourself to

Be here now with whatever is.

When practicing autogenics, each suggestion is repeated three times and the entire exercise itself needs to be repeated at three different periods each day. The best times are generally just before you get out of bed, just before you go to sleep, and at some time during the day. If there is no possibility of lying down during the day to repeat the exercise you can always do it sitting up in a chair. If you are in public draw your fists up to your chest by bending your elbows rather than bringing the whole arm above the head. Before long even the simple suggestion "My right arm is heavy" will trigger the psychophysical relaxation process in the whole body.

Some people get feelings of heaviness and warmth immediately; for others it takes as long as a week or two of practicing three times a day for ten or fifteen minutes at a time. But for everyone it comes eventually and with it a profound sense of relaxation. At the end of the series of self-directed instructions, *canceling* the training session occurs when you clench your hand into a fist and raise your arm straight above your head, or bend your arm and draw your fist to your shoulders, at the same time taking a deep breath and then stretching. This brings about an immediate return to normal consciousness although the temporary excursion into the realms of deep relaxation that you have just experienced continues to exercise benefits.

AUTOGENIC TRAINING MADE SIMPLE

With both eyes closed, repeat the following suggestions, each one three times:

- My left arm is heavy . . . My right arm is heavy
- Both arms are heavy . . . Both legs are heavy
- Arms and legs heavy . . . Arms and legs warm
- Breathing calm and easy . . . My heartbeat calm and easy
- My solar plexus is warm . . . My forehead is cool
- I am at peace

The return:

- Clench both fists
- Take a deep breath
- Flex both arms up in a stretch
- Breathe out slowly
- Return arms to sides
- Unclench fists
- Open your eyes
- Lie for a moment with eyes open
- Be here now with whatever is

Mind mystery

Just why such a simple mental exercise should bring about such profound benefits is at least a partial mystery. The neurophysiological mechanism by which the autonomic nervous system is controlled is by no means completely understood. But practicing autogenic training triggers you into a state of passive concentration that lets your mind and body work together toward more harmonious functioning.

CHAPTER 4

Go Free

Arriving home from a long day's work can be the lowest point in your day. You stagger through the front door, sigh with relief, and suddenly realize how overwrought you feel. A constant flow of adrenaline and the things you have had to do have kept you going all day, but now you're ready to collapse with nervous exhaustion. Perhaps you go straight to the refrigerator and begin sampling snack after snack—hoping eventually to find the magic food that will calm and restore you. Or you may collapse in front of the television and sit through a program you hate because you haven't got the energy to change the channel. Now you know you don't have to do this.

Stretch Out after Work

Some people find that half an hour's aerobic exercise straight after work is just what they need to shake off work-time worries and supply a new burst of energy. If aerobic exercise seems too energetic, try the stretch routines—a few simple stretches that rely mainly on the forces of gravity—so that all you do is let go and breathe. There's no jumping around or forcing your fatigued body to do umpteen situps. You'll be surprised how much doing these simple exercises for a few minutes a day can improve both the way you look and feel.

These stretching exercises should not be done right after a meal, as they may interfere with digestion. Choose a time when you can be alone to enjoy them and relax. If you like, stretch to the sound of gentle music.

Repeat this series of stretches every day, or choose one or two to do whenever you feel tense in a certain area.

Wall Presses

These exercises use the force of gravity and a wall to stretch out the muscles of your neck, shoulders, back, legs, and ankles.

Shoulder press

Stand three to four feet from a wall, arms shoulder width apart, and place your hands against the wall two feet above your head. Lean on your hands, letting your head and neck drop forward and your chest sink downward so that your back is bowed. Rotate the upper arms gently so that you don't hunch your shoulders. The stretch should last about thirty seconds.

Upper back press

Stand in the same position, and lift up your head and buttocks so that your back arches. Press the elbows toward the wall. Again, work the stretch for thirty seconds.

Heel, calf, and hip press

Stand about one foot away from the wall and put your arms straight out in front of you, level with your shoulders, and your hands against the wall. Place one foot back about two feet and press the heel toward the ground. You should feel the muscles in the back of your calf and heel stretch. By tilting your pelvis forward you can also stretch the front of your hip. After thirty seconds, change to the other leg.

Wall splits

Sit on the floor parallel to the wall, legs
extended in front of you, with one hip against
the wall. Now lie down, swinging both legs up
in an arc along the wall as you turn your body
around so that you end up in a V shape. Let
your legs fall gently open with the force of
gravity as far as is comfortable. (As you relax
into the stretch and exhale they will open
wider.) Extend your arms out to the sides parallel to the wall and allow your whole back to
widen and lengthen against the floor. Stay in
the stretch for two to three minutes and then
gently roll out of it.

Floor Work

Twist-overs

Lie on your back on the floor with your knees
bent. Take a few easy breaths and feel your
back lengthening. Cross your legs, left over
right, and tuck your left foot under your right
calf. Extend your arms out to the sides. Now
slowly drop your knees over to touch the floor
on the right side. Turn your head to the left.
Stretch out your left arm and try to get your
shoulder to reach the floor. Continue for thirty
to sixty seconds and then return knees to

center. Hug them into your chest with your arms to relax your lower back. Repeat the exercise on the other side and then repeat both sides again.

Lie back thigh stretch

Kneel on the floor, sitting back on your heels. Unless you are very supple, place a cushion or two behind you to lie on; with practice you may be able to remove the cushions and lie back on the floor. Move your legs apart to create a space to sit in, but don't worry if you can't sit right down between your legs. Place your hands behind you and gradually walk them backward. Gradually ease yourself further down, supporting yourself on your hands or forearms and making sure that your pelvis is tilted forward so that you don't strain your lower back.

Neck rocking

This is a good preparation for the yoga plow position, which otherwise can be a little uncomfortable if you go into it without this warm-up. Kneel down and rest the top of your head on the floor in front of you. Gently rock forward and backward over your scalp, feeling the stretch in your neck and upper back. Continue the exercise for one minute.

The plow

Lie on your back. You may want to place a rolled-up hand towel or sweater under your neck for comfort. Bring your knees up to your chest and extend your legs up toward the ceiling. Allow your legs to drop over your head and let the weight of gravity bring them gradually down. The aim is to drop your feet all the way to the floor behind your head. Continue the stretch for one minute and then slowly roll your legs back down again, feeling each vertebra roll against the floor. Rest for a moment, lengthening out your spine along the floor, then repeat the stretch.

Roll–up

Assume a crouching position with your feet comfortably apart, dropping your heels as close to the ground as possible. Hang in this position for thirty seconds, then place your hands on the floor in front of you and lift your bottom up toward the ceiling, straightening your legs if possible, but not straining. When your legs are straight, gradually roll up through the spine until you are standing. Stand tall and take a few deep breaths, feeling the relaxation in your muscles and in the ease of your posture.

Bath Bliss

In a world where the benefits of an invigorating quick shower are more and more appreciated, it is easy to forget the bliss and stress-relieving potential of a long lazy bath. Water—especially when it has been fortified with plant essences—has the power to soothe, heal, and relax a tense body and to lift a fatigued spirit.

Mind-potions

Allow an hour for the whole process from beginning to end. Make sure you have everything you need—towel, loofah or hemp glove, and another towel to use as a headrest. Add essential oils to the water as the bath is filling, using about ten to fifteen drops total of either a single essence or of a mixture for a large bath. Each essence has a different effect on the mind and body. Let them work their wonders while you carry out a relaxing and waste-eliminating self-massage. When your bath is finished, lie down for ten minutes with an eye mask or a piece of dark fabric across your eyes and keep warm.

The massage message

Water is the perfect medium for self-massage.
The heat of the water works silent wonders and
the water supports your body so that you have
easy access to feet, legs, arms, and torso while
still remaining relaxed. When you get into the
bath, gently scrub yourself all over with a hemp
glove or a loofah. Then just relax and soak for a
few minutes, letting the heat penetrate your
muscles. Keep a cool cloth nearby to smooth
over your face when needed.

Now you are ready for massage, which is
nothing more than stroking, kneading, pushing,
and pressing your skin and muscles. Start with
your feet. Grasp one foot between thumb and
fingers and press in between the tendons,
gently at first, then harder and harder, moving
from the toes up toward the ankle. Then, using
your fingertips and knuckles, go over the soles
of your feet. Wherever you find a sore spot,
work harder until you feel the discomfort melt
beneath your hand. Now do your heel, grasping
it between thumb and fingers and working
around the area of the Achilles tendon. This is
also a good time to make circles with your foot
to loosen the ankle joint. Repeat this with
the other foot and then go on to your legs.

Lift each leg in turn and deeply stroke the
flesh on the back, from the ankle up to the

knee. Then go back to the ankle again and repeat the same motions on the side and front of the calf. Keep working and, as you massage a little deeper with each stroke, you will gradually find that any tautness softens. Now go over your thighs with the same movement and afterward knead and squeeze around the knee area wherever there are trouble spots, just as you did on the feet. Now knead each thigh and hip, then go on to your arms.

Knead and squeeze every spot you can reach on your shoulders and neck, looking for sore spots and focusing on the areas between joints and muscles. Pay particular attention to the tops of the shoulders, where most of us lock away our tension. Grasp this area in your thumb and fingers and insistently ease away any hardness you find there. Finally, go over your ribs, doing each side with its opposite hand.

ESSENCE ALCHEMY

As part of the benevolent bath, choose essential oils not so much for what they can do for your skin as what they can do to expand your consciousness and lift your spirit. Whatever your mental state may be, it has an enchanting antidote from the world of flowers.

Negative State	Essential Oil Remedy
anger	ylang ylang, rose, chamomile
resentment	rose
sadness	hyssop, marjoram, sandalwood
mental fatigue	basil, peppermint, cypress, patchouli
worry	lavender
feeling jaded	neroli, melissa, camphor
feelings of weakness	chamomile, jasmine, melissa
irritability	frankincense, marjoram, lavender, chamomile
physical exhaustion	jasmine, rosemary, juniper, patchouli
anxiety	sage, juniper, basil, jasmine

Forget Insomnia

A lot of so-called insomnia is nothing more than the result of worrying about getting to sleep. Many people who consider themselves insomniacs are really victims of the general propaganda about sleep rather than true nonsleepers. Many people seek treatment because they can only sleep four or five hours a night, although that may be all they need. There is nothing more likely to cause sleeplessness than the worry that you won't be able to drop off. Sometimes sleeplessness can be normal. After all, we all experience a sleepless night now and then, particularly if we are overtired, worried, or excited about some coming event.

How—and How Not—to Get to Sleep

Next time you are troubled by sleeplessness take a look at nature's sleep aids.

* Get more exercise regularly during the day. This helps burn up stress-caused adrenaline buildup in the brain, which can result in that tense, nervous feeling that you are "up" and can't seem to get "down." Don't engage in strenuous exercise just before going to bed as

it can set the heart pounding and stimulate the whole body too much.

- Don't go to bed when you are not sleepy. Instead, pursue some pleasant activity, preferably passive. Television is not the best choice, for radiation emitted from the set can disturb your nervous system when you least need it.

- Don't drink coffee, alcohol, or strong stimulants at dinner. This isn't just an old wives' tale. Alcohol may put you to sleep but it tends not to keep you there, awakening you instead in the early hours of the morning.

- Try some *Passiflora*. Passionflower is one of the world's best natural tranquilizers. It is readily available in the form of tablets that you can take before bed or when you need a "downer" and it is not habit-forming as are many other tranquilizers.

- Drink milk. It is an old-fashioned remedy, maybe, but it is a scientifically sound assertion that drinking a glass of milk before bed helps you to sleep. Milk contains tryptophan, a precursor to one of the calming brain chemicals called serotonin, which is important for relaxation and for inducing sleep.

- Use an ionizer. This is a little contraption put beside your bed that sends negative ions into the air and is a godsend to anyone who has the kind of nervous system that tends to go "up" and doesn't want to come "down."

- Get into a rut. Go to bed as much as possible at the same time every night and develop a routine or simple ritual about it. Doing the same thing every night before going to bed quickly accustoms the mind to accept sleep.

- Write your troubles away. If you have trouble with a racing mind, rather than trying to block all your thoughts, face them. Take a pen and some paper and write down all the things that come into your mind. When you run out of things to write, assure yourself that you can let go of all those concerns for the night because they will be right there on the paper when you wake up.

- An excellent hydrotherapy technique is to take a pair of cotton socks and soak them with cold water. Wring them out well and put them on your feet. Cover the socks with a second pair of dry ones—either wool or cotton—and retire for the night.

- Listen to mellow music. Music can help alter consciousness and have you sinking blissfully into the depths of slumber.

- Some of the essential plant oils have a wonderful calming effect on the mind and body. You can take a warm bath with them or place a few drops on your pillow to inhale through the night. For the bath use four drops of lavender oil, two drops of camomile, and two drops of neroli (orange blossom). Or try a drop or two of each on your pillow.

- Begin each day with twenty minutes in the sun or in very bright light. Your circadian rhythms are linked to sunlight. The sun sets our natural clocks properly and acts as a natural energizer, too.

- Learn to breathe deeply. It is amazingly tranquilizing and the best possible antidote to anxiety.

- Practice a relaxation or meditation technique twice a day. A valuable tool for sleeplessness, it will lower elevated blood pressure and help you cope better with whatever stress you tend to carry off to bed with you.

- Tranquility teas can help. Get to know the natural tranquilizers and herb teas, and whenever you feel the need, use them, sweetened with honey if you like, as a bedtime drink. Peppermint, camomile, skullcap, catnip, and vervain are renowned for their relaxing effects.

Stop worrying about getting to sleep. Just let it happen. If it doesn't tonight, so what? It will tomorrow night. Or the next. Lack of sleep is not going to kill you, but worrying about it for long enough just might.

Make Stress Work for You

Learning to make stress work for you rather than against you can unlock new ways of responding to what happens at home, at work, and in relationships with the rest of the world. Once you make a friend of stress, forces that once seemed to be working against you become positive energies that define you, strengthen you, and help you express your own brand of creativity and joy.

Further Reading

If you benefited from this book by health and beauty expert Leslie Kenton, you might like to try the entire series of quick and easy tips for living:

BEAT STRESS (8041-1719-5)
Discover how to identify, then eliminate everyday tension through relaxation, diet, and exercise.

BOOST ENERGY (8041-1720-9)
Increase your stamina and optimize your efficiency by changing your everyday routine.

GET FIT (8041-1721-7)
Develop the best exercise program for your lifestyle, and find out how to stick with it.

LOOK GREAT (8041-1722-5)
Learn the basics for making the most of your
appearance by selecting, or creating, effective
beauty products.

LOSE FAT (8041-1723-3)
Win the weight war through a simple eating
plan that turns food into energy—not fat.

SLEEP DEEP (8041-1724-1)
Get the rest you need with relaxation techniques and healthy, natural sleep potions.

Index

SPONTANEOUS HEALING
by Andrew Weil, M.D.

The best medicine does not merely combat germs or suppress symptoms, but rather works hand in hand with the body's natural defenses to manage illness. Drawing on fascinating case histories from his own practice as well as medical techniques he has observed in his world travels, Dr. Weil shows how spontaneous healing has worked to resolve life-threatening diseases, severe trauma, and chronic pain.

DR. DEAN ORNISH'S PROGRAM
FOR REVERSING
HEART DISEASE
by Dr. Dean Ornish

Dr. Dean Ornish is the first clinician to offer documented proof that heart disease can be halted or even reversed simply by changing your lifestyle. In this breakthrough book, he guides you step-by-step through the extraordinary Opening Your Heart Program that takes you beyond the purely physical side of health care to include the psychological, emotional, and spiritual aspects so vital to healing.

FOOD AND HEALING
by Annemarie Colbin

We must take responsibility for our own health and rely less on modern medicine, which seems to focus on trying to cure rather than prevent illness. Eating well is the first step toward better health and includes the latest information on new dietary systems, low-fat eating, food combining, and alternative medicine.

BETWEEN HEAVEN AND EARTH:
A Guide to Chinese Medicine
by Harriet Beinfield, L. Ac.,
and
Efrem Korngold, L. Ac., O.M.D.

Pioneers in the practice of acupuncture and herbal medicine explain the philosophy behind Chinese medicine, how it works, and what it can do. Combining Eastern traditions with Western sensibilities in a unique blend that is relevant today, this book addresses three vital areas of Chinese medicine to present a comprehensive yet understandable guide to this ancient system.

NATURAL PRESCRIPTIONS
by Robert M. Giller, M.D., and
Kathy Matthews

A natural treatment is the best kind—one that helps the body heal itself. Based on his years of practical experience as a doctor, as well as on the latest research, Dr. Giller's book explains in crystal-clear terms how to treat yourself with vitamin and mineral supplements, herbs, diet, exercise, and stress reduction.